Desserts

The Cann Family
and

Yummy

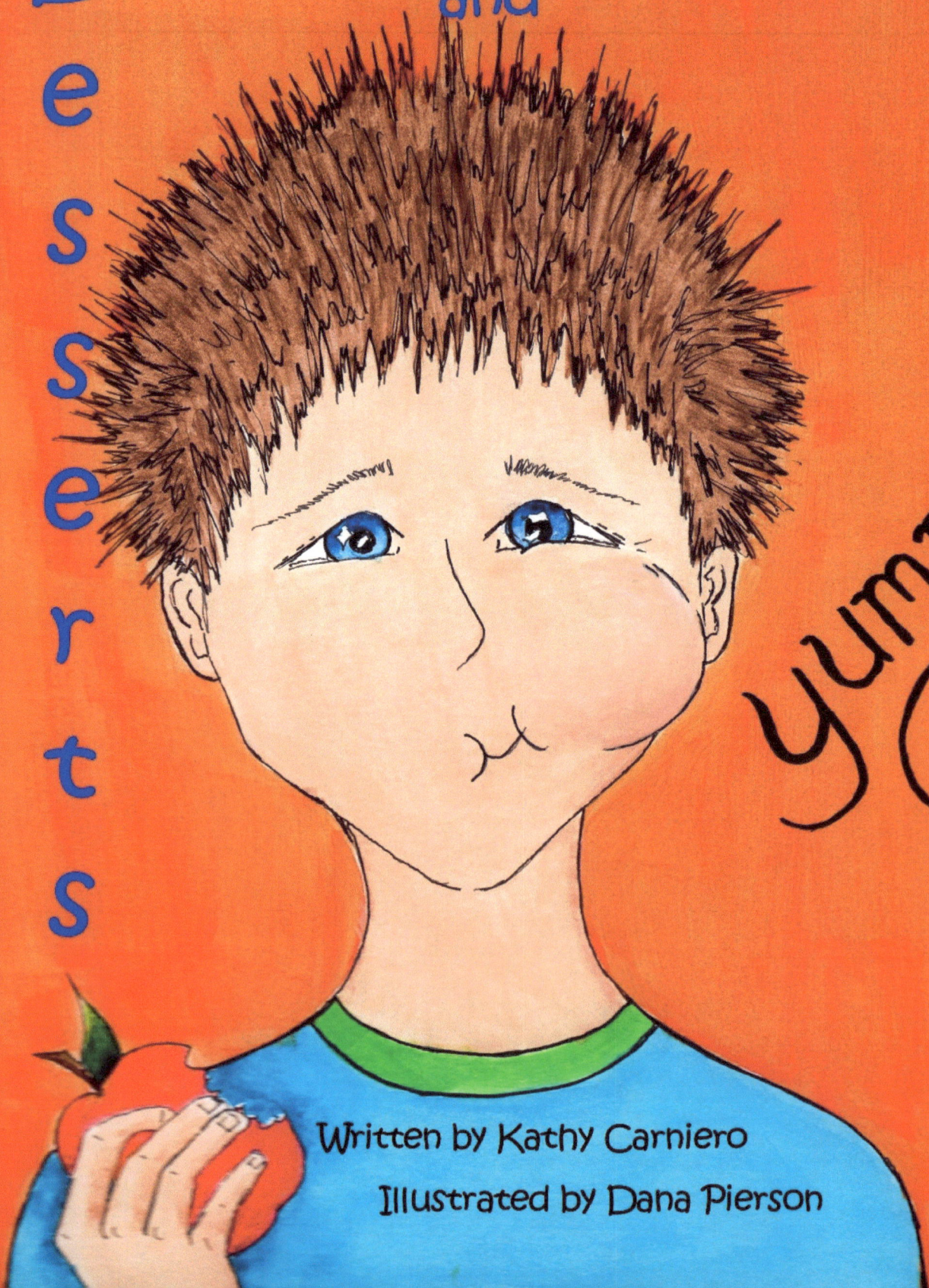

Written by Kathy Carniero

Illustrated by Dana Pierson

Published by Live Love Learn Books Publishing

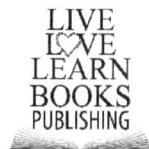

LIVE
LOVE
LEARN
BOOKS
PUBLISHING

The Cann Family and Desserts Copyright © 2014 Kathy Carniero

All rights reserved.

Cover art and illustrations designed by Dana Pierson.

Printed in the United States of America

ISBN-10: 0990304418

ISBN-13: 978-0-9903044-1-8

Library of Congress Control Number: 2014920996

This book is dedicated to Anthony, Irelynn, Raelynn

Haley, Ethan, and Hanna

Hope you enjoy!

From The Cann Family

to your family!

As the moon disappeared and the sun began to shine over the Cann's house, mom Amy, dad Paul, brother Zander and sister Lillian were all snuggled in their beds. Zander the oldest, woke up first from his nights sleep full of colorful dreams and far off places.

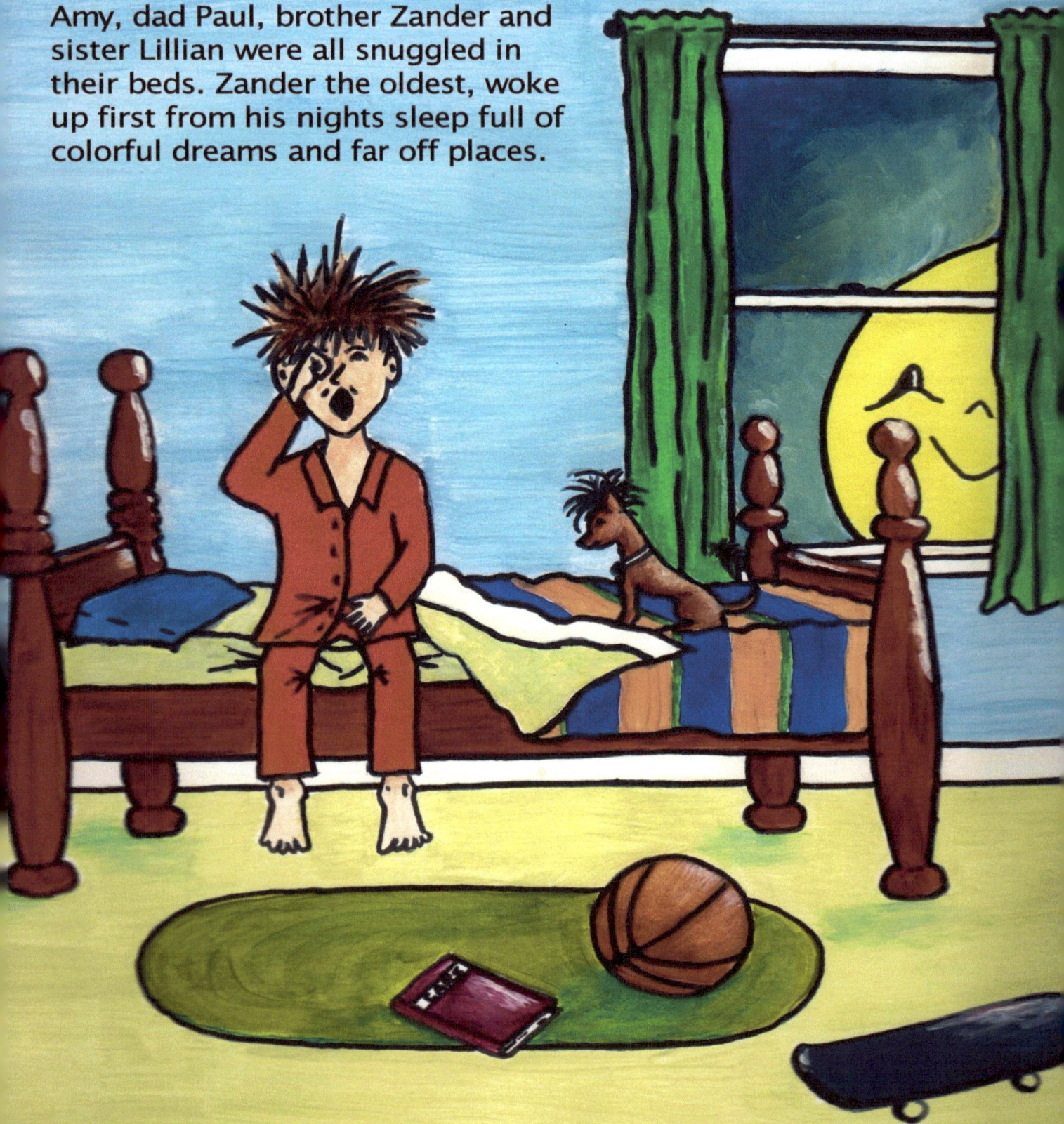

He quickly got dressed and ran down stairs. Amy had woken up too and was in the kitchen enjoying her morning coffee. "Good morning mom!" Zander happily sang out. "Good morning sunshine" His mom said sweetly.

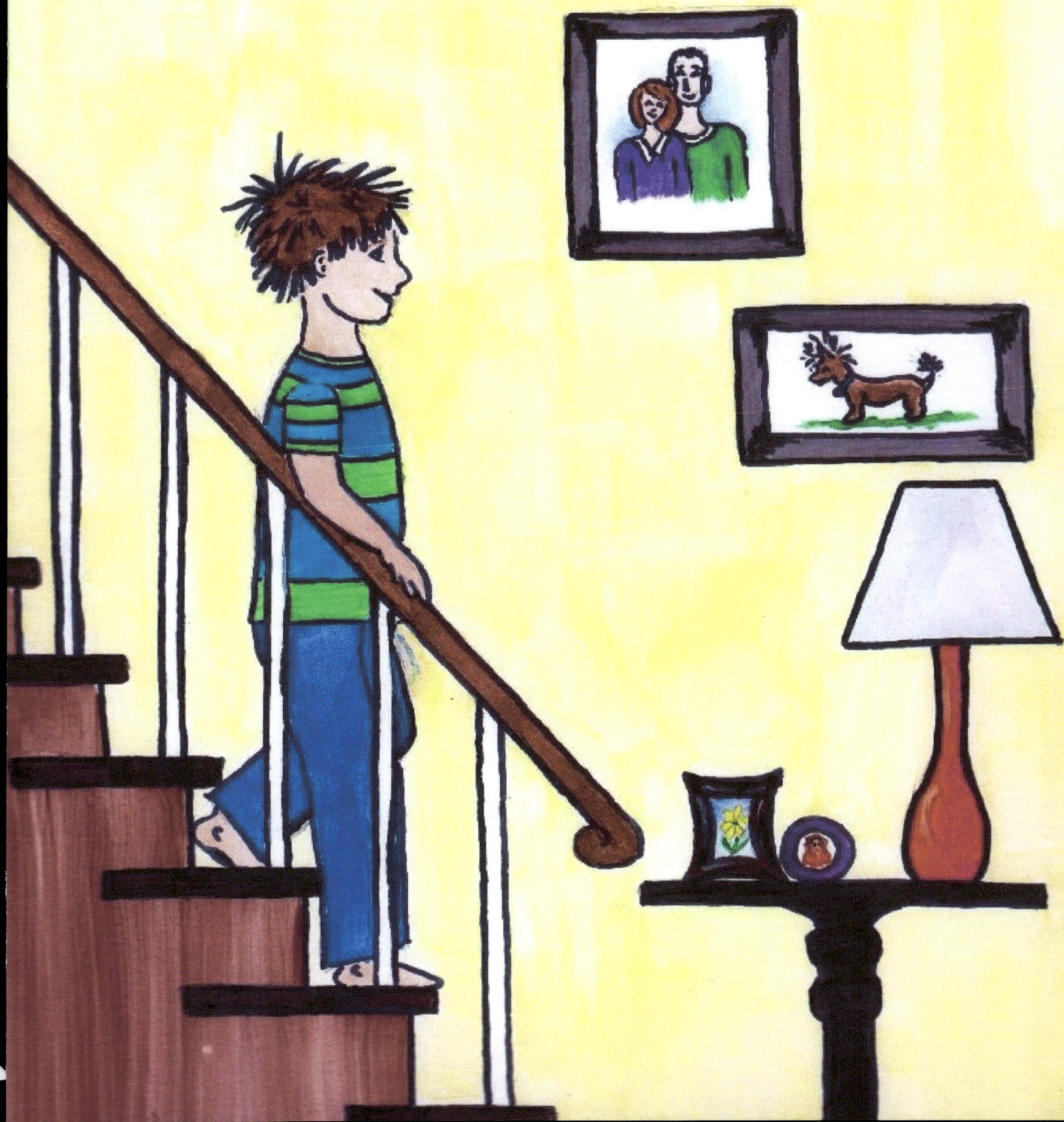

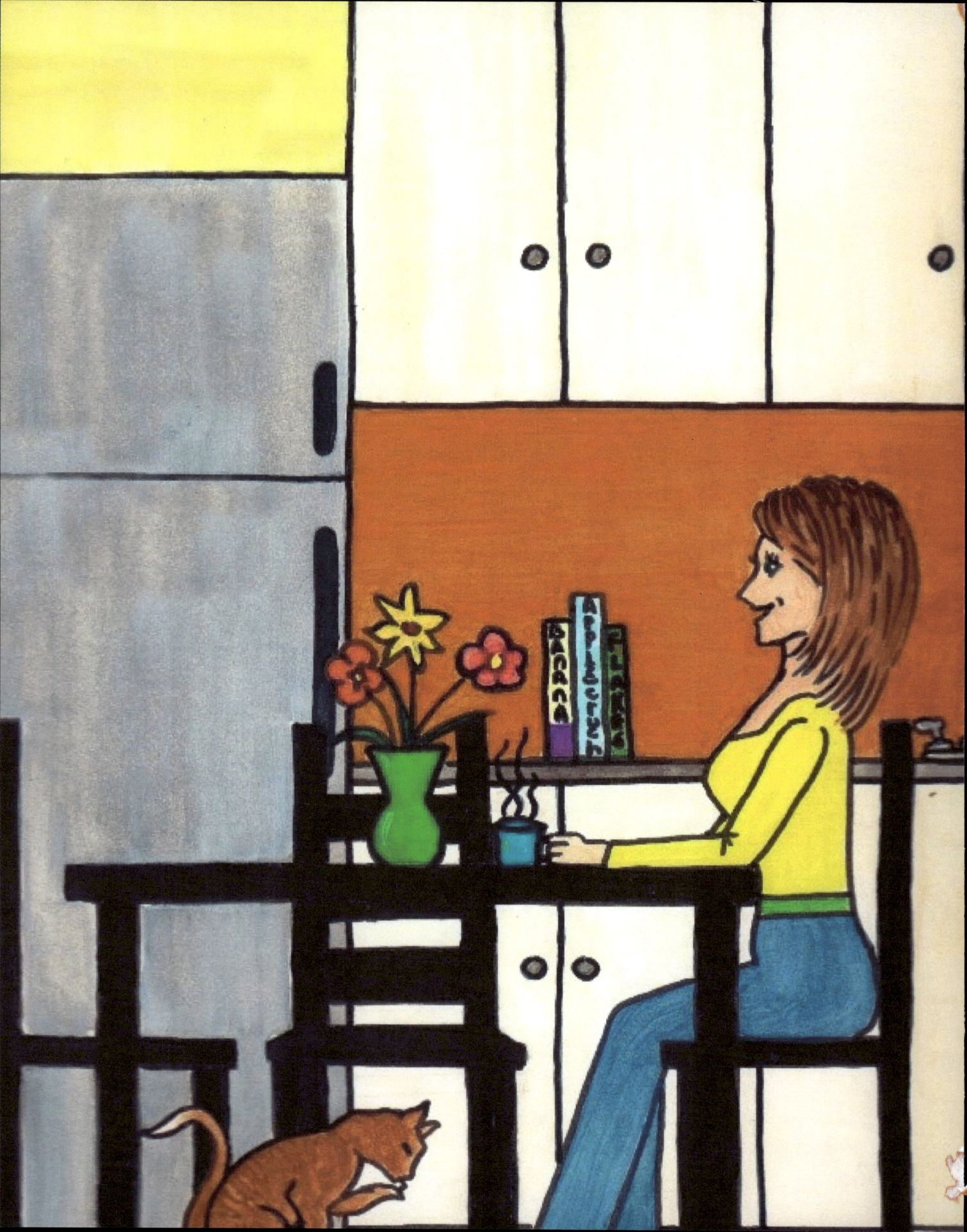

"Mom, I have a great idea! You and I should go to the store and get Lillian and I some yummy desserts to eat after dinner tonight."

"That is a great idea Zander! Let me finish my coffee and we will go before Lillian and daddy wake up. We can surprise them!" She shouted with excitement.

The two got ready and headed to the nearest store.

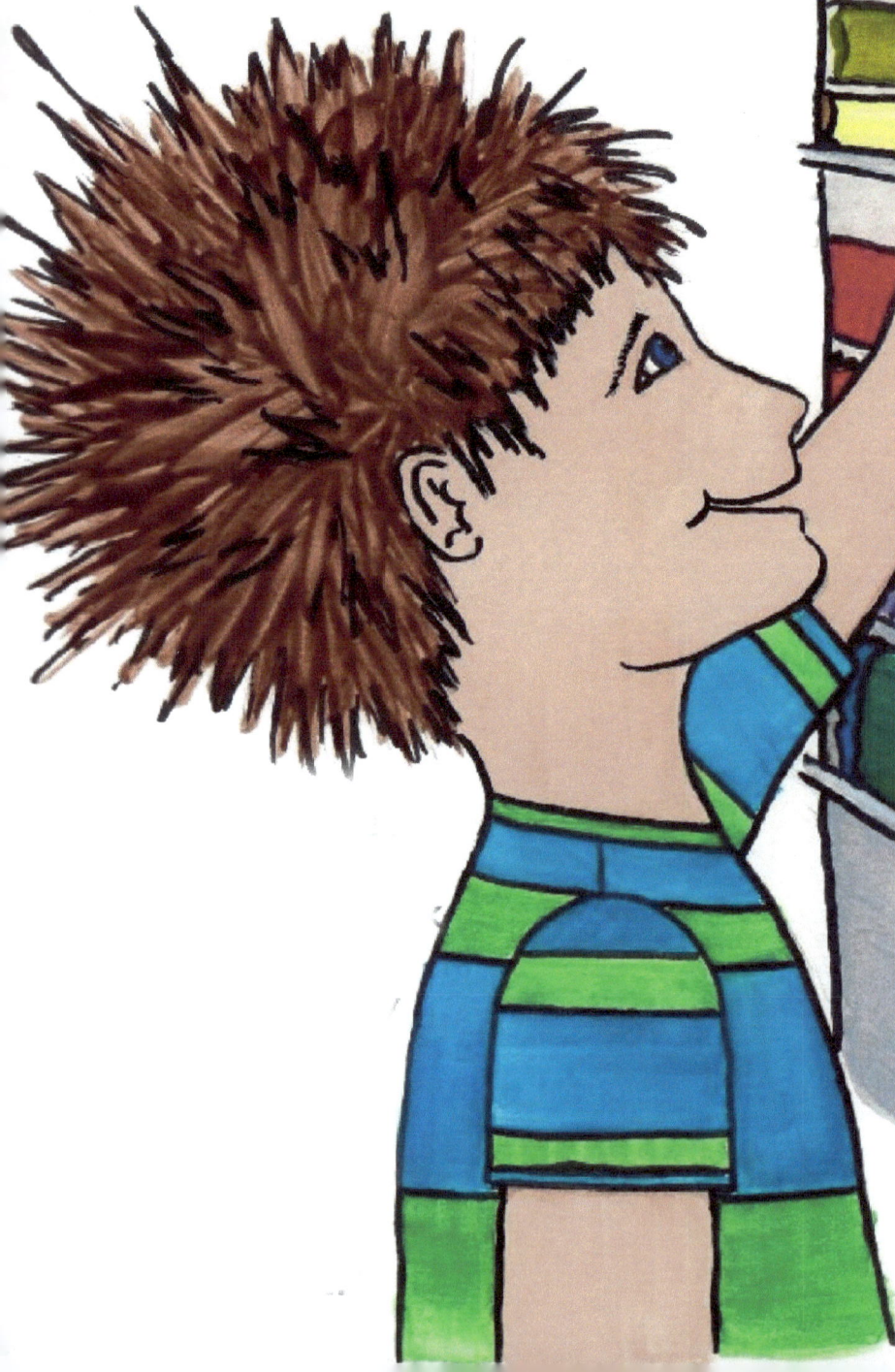

As soon as they got inside Zander ran straight to the cookie aisle. "So much to choose from" he said to himself. He grabbed the brightest and yummiest looking bag of cookies he could find.

Zander started to go to the next aisle when out of no where he ehard this tiny voice. "Hey you! Down here!" Squeaked the tiny voice. Zander looked down at his bag of cookies and saw they were talking to him!

"Well hello cookies!" Zander said. The cookies replied back sadly, "I know we look really yummy and our bag is bright and shiny, but we are really not the best choice for your dessert tonight."

"What do you mean?" Zander asked confused. "Well," Cookies said, "unlike our good friend the apple, us cookies are full of sugars and fats that will not help you grow big and strong, we can make you weak, cause you to be tired and give you cavities. Please put us back and go meet our friend."

"Ok!" Zander said. As he put the cookies back he thought to himself. Those cookies are right, they may taste really good, but I want to grow big and strong. I wonder what their apple friend has to say.

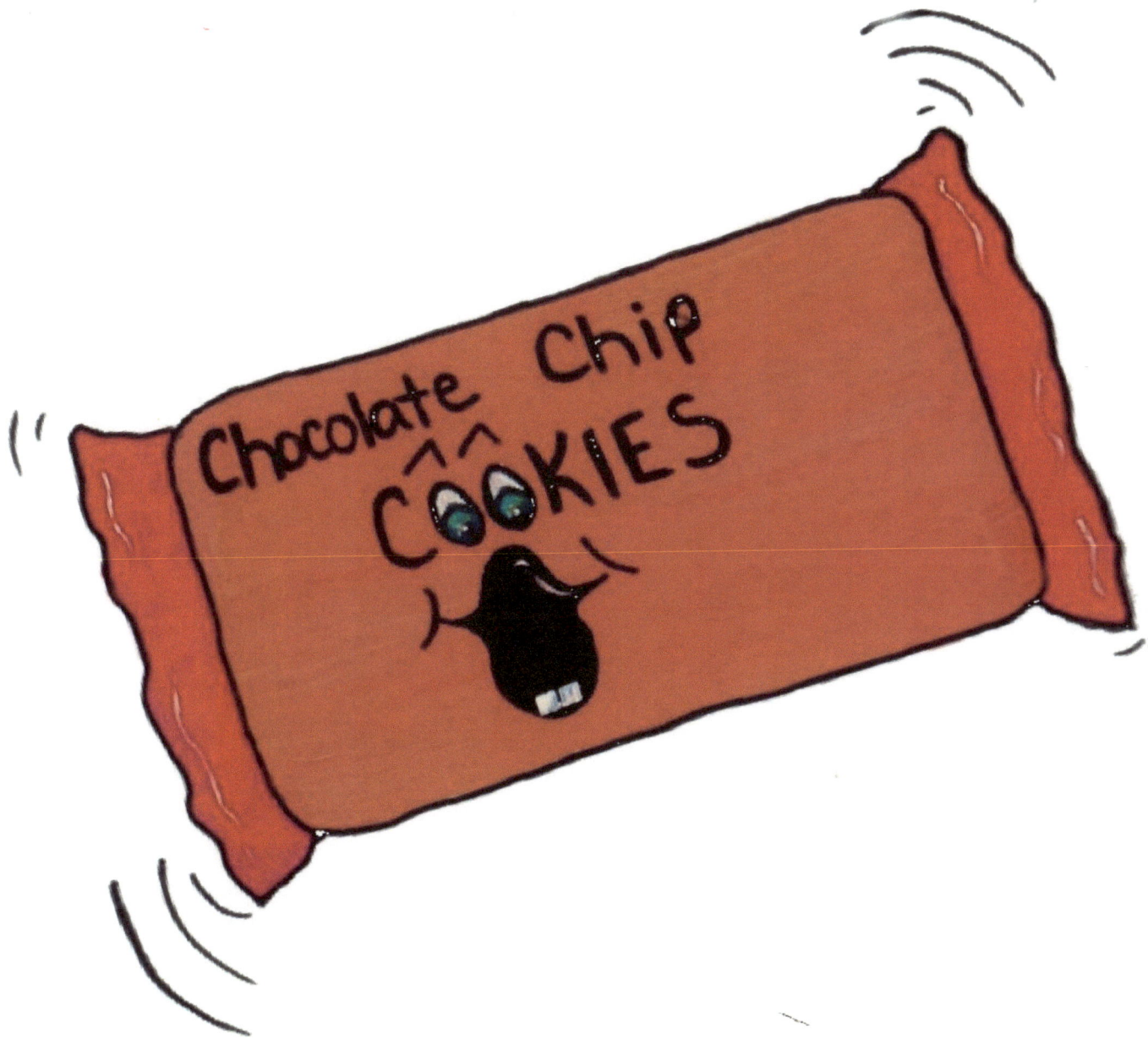

Zander made his way over to the fruit aisle and picked up a shiny red apple. "Hi there Apple! I just met your friend Cookies and he told me to come pick you for my dessert tonight."

"Oh yepeee!" The apple shouted. "Yes, unlike our friend Cookies, us Apples help you grow strong and stay healthy. Ever hear someone say, an apple a day keeps the doctor away? That is because we are full of the important daily vitamins A, B, C, E and K. These vitamins help keep you healthy on the inside and outside of your body. When you eat us, we also help keep your teeth clean. We come in fun colors like red, yellow, and green. We can taste sweet or sour, and you can even dip us in your favorite yogurt! After you choose us, please go meet our other friend the banana."

Zander was so excited to have chosen a dessert that will not only taste good, but will help him stay healthy too.

He now made his way over to the bananas.

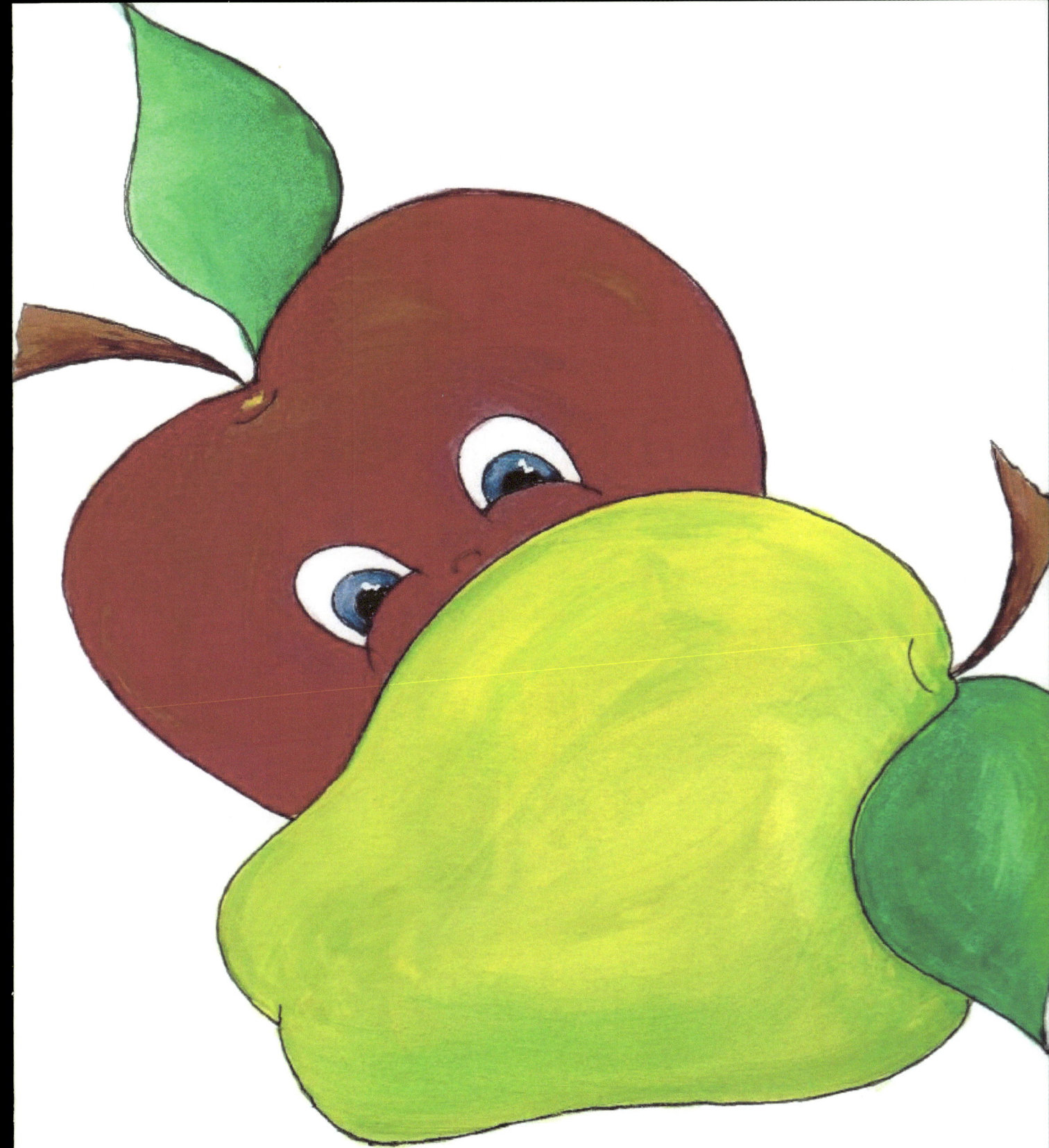

"Hello there Bananas!" Zander shouted.
"I just chose your friend the apple for my dessert
  tonight, are y"all good too?"

   The bananas were so excited Zander had come over
to them. "Of course we are!" They shouted, "and unlike
our friend Cookies and their cousin Chips who are full
of bad sugars, fats, and preservatives that are not good
for you. We are full of vitamins and nutrition.
Did you know that we even have a special mineral in
us called potassium? This mineral helps to build your
muscles, and keeps your brain and heart healthy!
We are also fun to eat just like the apples, you can slice
us up and put us in cereal, or just peel our peel
and enjoy our soft sweet taste. Choose us and then
please go over and meet our other friend the carrots."

   Zander was even more excited now knowing
he was choosing desserts that were going
to be good for him and Lillian. He put the bananas
next to the apples and walked over to meet Carrots.

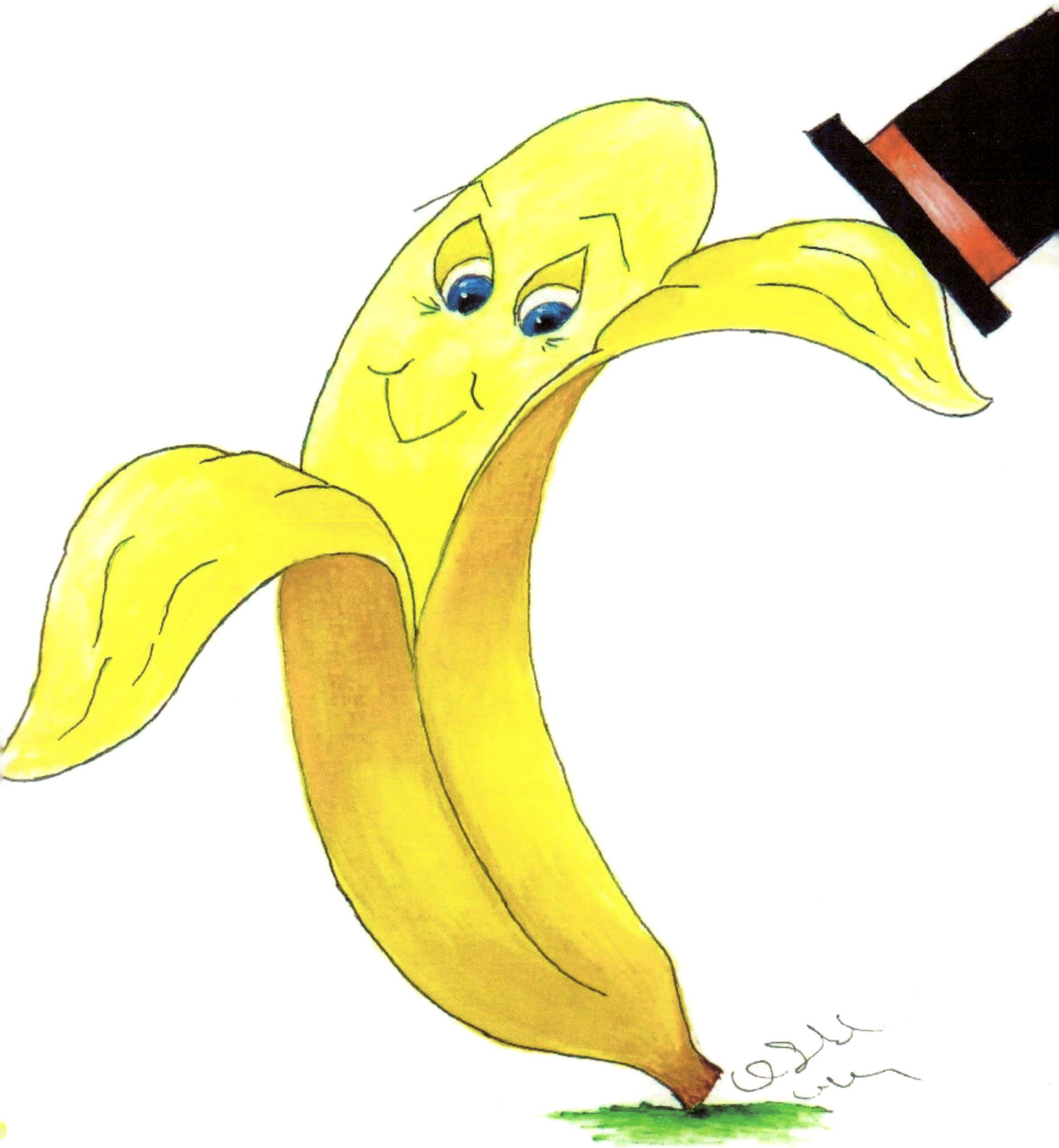

"Nice to meet you Carrots!" Zander said, but the carrots did not talk back. Hhhhmmm......
Zander thought, this is strange. He picked up the carrots and said to them again. "Nice to meet you Carrots!" Still nothing. He then decided to shake them a bit when all of a sudden the carrots started to yell. "What's going on out there? Can't you see we are sleeping here?" "Well," Zander said. "I just met your friends Apples and Bananas. I have chosen them for my dessert tonight instead of Cookies and Chips. They told me to come meet you too."

"Really!" The carrots screeched. Then sadly they whispered, "all we do is sleep over here because no one ever chooses us anymore. They always want to choose our other friends Cake and Candy Bar, and just like their friends Cookies and cousin Chips, they are also full of bad sugars, fats, preservatives and processed ingredients that are bad for you. Us Carrots are high in vitamin A which your body needs to help strengthen your skin, eyes, teeth and bones. With out us, you will not have the right nutrition to stay strong and healthy. We know we look kind of funny, but we are crunchy and taste sweet. You can even dip us in ranch dressing! Yummy!" They shouted with excitement.

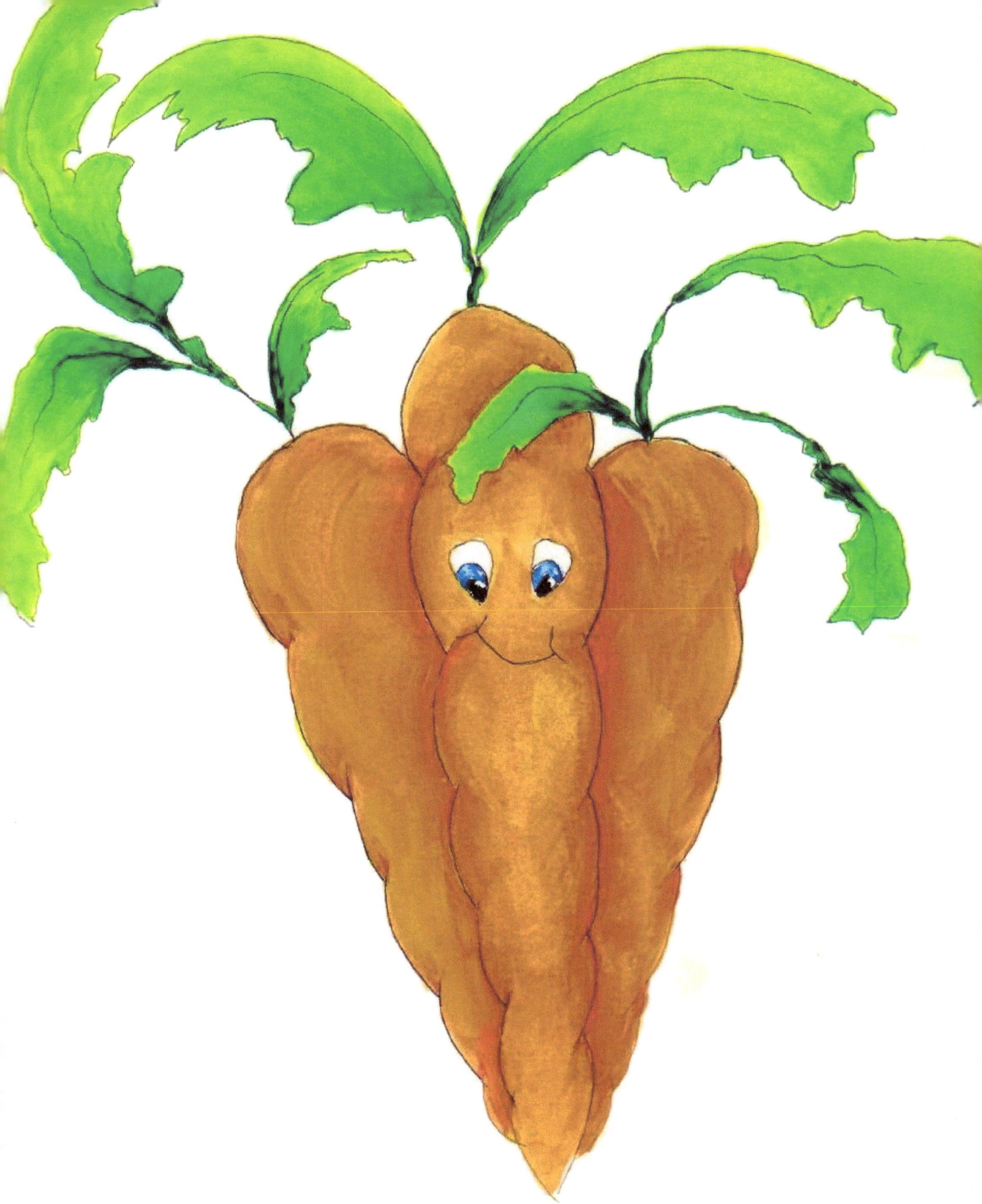

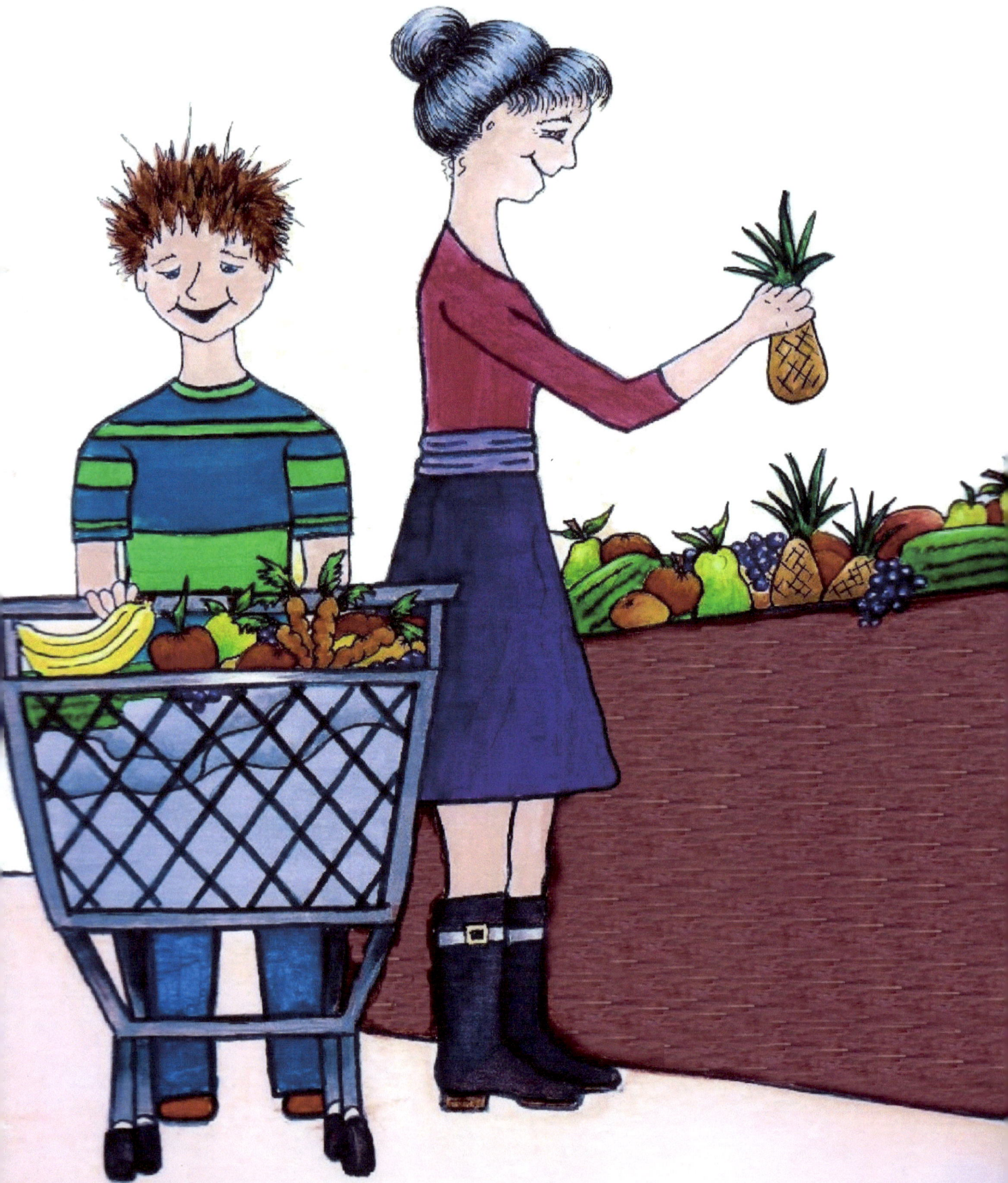

With a huge grin on his face Zander put the
carrots in his basket along with the apples
and bananas.

As he made his way over to meet his mom
at the check out he grabbed some ranch dressing,
yogurt and cereal. "Look mom"! He shouted. He
showed his mom the desserts and told her how
he learned they were good for him.

Amy felt very proud of her son for making
the right dessert choices.

As they drove back home Zander couldn't wait to tell his dad Paul and sister Lillian about the yummy and healthy desserts they were going to have tonight.

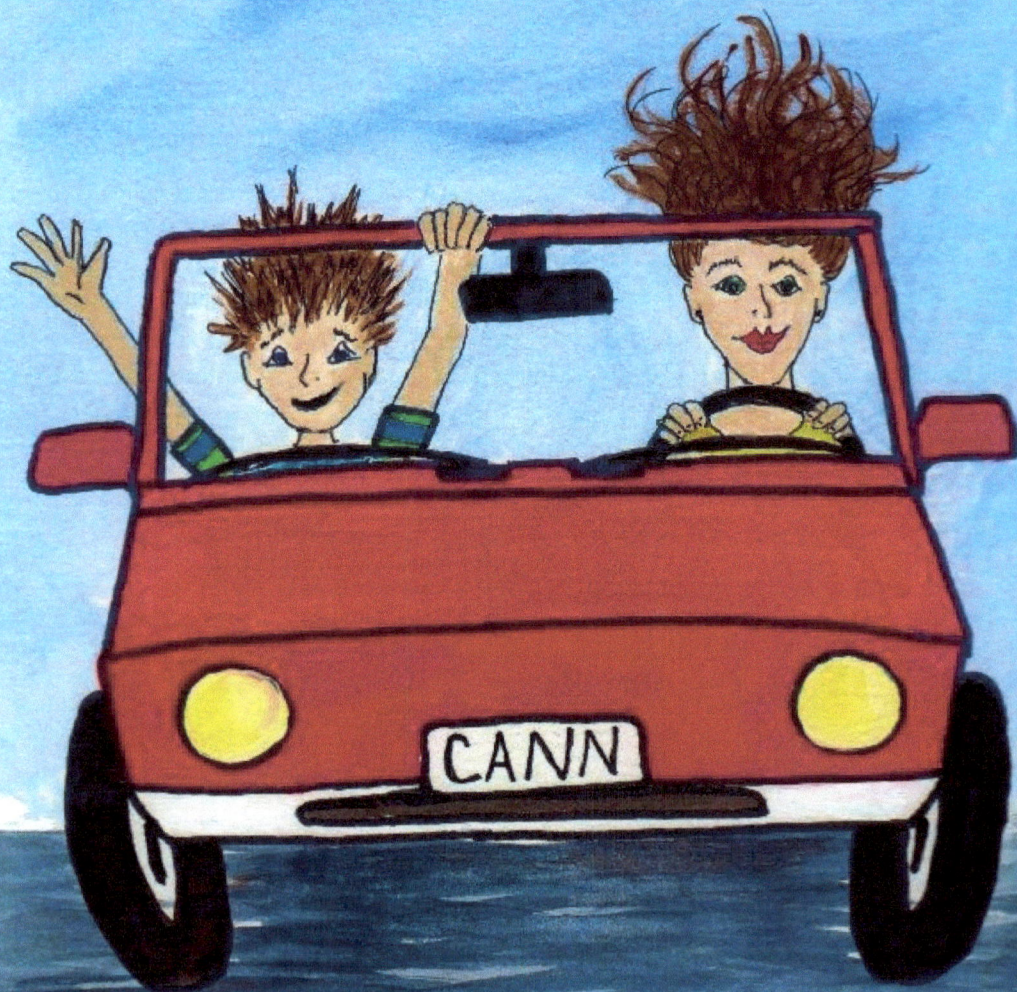

"If the Cann family can choose healthy desserts, so can your family!"

Family Project

Parents and kids can make healthier dessert choices together. As a family make a list of all the healthy desserts you can choose at the store. Write down all the fun and creative ways you and your family can enjoy these desserts. This will make your trip to the grocery store fun and adventurous.
Happy healthy eating from the Cann family!

List

_____

_____

_____

_____

_____

The End

About the Author

Kathy Carniero lives in a small town outside of Dallas Tx.

She is the mother to three fun, crazy and loving kids.

In her spare time Kathy enjoys spending time with her husband and family.

Kathy knows how important it is to teach children

about life's ups and downs and learn how to overcome challenges.

She also knows how hard it can be,

and that is why The Cann Family books were created.

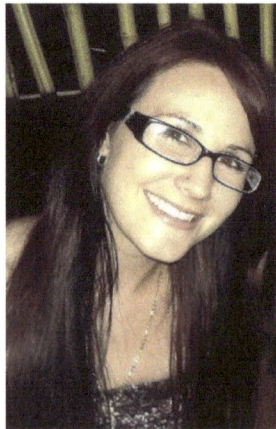

About the Illustrator

Dana lives in a small town outside of Dallas, TX.

As a self-taught artist she is naturally talented and gifted.

She has been drawing and painting since she was a teenager.

Adding to her creativity, Dana has begun designing and making earrings.

Dana has two daughters and 6 grandkids.

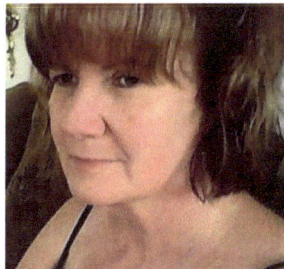

www.ingramcontent.com/pod-product-compliance
Lightning Source LLC
Chambersburg PA
CBHW042118040426
42449CB00002B/97